SHEPHERDING A CHILD'S HEART

LEADER'S GUIDE

by Bill Hill

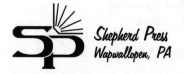
Shepherd Press
Wapwallopen, PA

©1999 by Bill Hill

ISBN 0-9663786-3-6

Unless otherwise noted, Scripture quotations are from the *New
International Version* (NIV), ©1994 International Bible Society. Italic text
indicates emphasis added.

Design and composition by Colophon Typesetting
Cover design by Tobias Outerwear for Books!

Manufactured in the United States of America

Contents

CONTENTS

Preface

It has been a great joy to see the response to *Shepherding a Child's Heart*. This joy is multi-faceted. Naturally one is pleased when his life's work is accepted and appreciated by the Body of Christ. Additionally it is a great joy to meet scores and scores of young people who are reading and appreciating the principles and perspective of *Shepherding a Child's Heart*. As I travel, I meet people who have been learning to shepherd their own hearts and the hearts of their children. A third facet of my joy is the insight and creativity of ministers of the gospel like Bill Hill, who have taken the things in *Shepherding a Child's Heart* and worked with them to make the truths in the book more accessible to others.

This leader's guide is designed to make sure that the things taught in *Shepherding a Child's Heart* are caught by the readers. Bill Hill has identified the important teaching in each section of the book and asked the appropriate questions to aid group leaders in being sure that others have understood the content of what they have read.

It is my hope that this leader's guide for *Shepherding a Child's Heart* will be a valuable tool for the faithful people who are taking study groups through the content of the book.

Tedd Tripp
July 1999

Introduction to the Leader's Guide

Shepherding a Child's Heart is the most helpful book I have read on the subject of child rearing. I have used it in my own parenting, with my school staff and with parents in my church and school. Tedd Tripp has done a masterful job at practically dealing with the theology of parenting. This study guide was designed to enable the leader to more efficiently extract the data of the book. It is not intended to take you beyond the content but to help you better assimilate, focus on and digest what the author is saying.

In an effort to best compliment Dr. Tripp's book, I have allowed the publisher to use the NIV translation in the Leader's Guide rather than the KJV translation, which was in the original Leader's Guide.

Bill Hill

Shepherding A Child's Heart

LEADER'S GUIDE

Introduction

1. *Today's parents are part of the generation that threw off authority. Give at least two results of the way that generation has impacted the culture.*
   A. It is no longer culturally acceptable for dad to be the "boss" at home.
   B. Mom doesn't obediently do what dad says.
   C. Dad, for his part, no longer lives in fear of the boss or of being fired through caprice. (p. xviii)

2. *What is the author's point for raising this issue?*
   A. Children raised in this climate no longer sit in neat rows at school.
   B. They no longer ask permission to speak.
   C. They no longer fear the results of talking back to their parents.
   D. In summary, they do not accept a submissive role in life. (p. xviii)

3. *In general, what ways have parents responded to this non-submission by the children?*
   A. Today's parents are frustrated and confused.
   B. Children don't act like they should and parents don't understand why.
   C. Many have concluded the job isn't possible
   D. Some simply turn away in frustration.
   E. Others keep trying to make the old John Wayne approach of the 1950's work. (p. xviii)

4. *In what capacity do you exercise authority as a parent?*
   As God's agent. (p. xix)

5. *Toward what two poles does our culture tend?*
   A. We tend toward a crass kind of John Wayne authoritarianism; or,
   B. We tend toward being a wimp. (p. xix)

6. *God calls you to exercise authority as a parent in what way?*
   Not in making your children do what you want, but in being true servants/authorities that lay down your lives. (p. xx)

7. *What is the purpose for the authority that you exercise in the lives of your children?*
   It is not to hold them under your power, but to empower them to be self-controlled people living freely under the authority of God. (p. xx)

8. *If authority best describes the parent's relationship to the child, then what describes the activity of the parent to the child?*
   "Shepherding" describes the activity of the parent to the child. The parent is the child's guide. (p. xx)

9. *Because your children desperately need to understand not only the external "what" they did wrong but also the internal "why" they did it, to what must your parenting goal not be limited?*
   Your parenting goal must not be limited to well behaved children. (p. xxi)

10. *In what direction does giving your children a keepable standard drive them?*
    Giving a keepable standard drives them away from the cross. (p. xxii)

Chapter One

Getting To The Heart Of Behavior

1. *List at least two truths about the heart taught in Proverbs 4:23; Mark 7:21; and Luke 6:45.*
   A. The heart is the control center for life. A person's life mirrors his heart.
   B. The heart determines behavior.
   C. Behavior is not the basic issue of child rearing. The basic issue is always what is going on in the heart. (pp. 3–4)

2. *What does Jesus call behavioral change that does not stem from a change in the heart?*
   Jesus calls behavioral change that is not from the heart "hypocrisy." In Matthew 15 Jesus denounces the Pharisees who honored him with their lips while their hearts were far from Him. Jesus censors them as people who wash the outside of the cup while the inside is still unclean. Yet this is what we often do in child rearing. We demand changed behavior and never address the heart that drives the behavior. (p. 4)

3. *What is the typical answer to a scenario in which two children are fighting over the same toy?*
   "Who had it first?" (p. 5)

4. *In what way does this typical answer miss the biblical mark?*
   This response misses heart issues. "Who had it first" is an issue of justice. Justice

operates in the favor of the child who is the quicker draw at getting the toy to begin with. (p. 5)

5. *When the above scenario is evaluated in terms of the heart, what issues change?*
    A. Now you have two offenders. Both children are displaying a hardness of heart toward the other. Both are being selfish. Both are saying "I don't care about you or your happiness."
    B. In terms of issues of the heart, you have two sinning children. Two children are preferring themselves before the other. Two children are breaking God's law. (pp. 5–6)

6. *To what is all behavior linked?*
    To some attitude of heart. (p. 6)

7. *List several things this understanding of the heart does for discipline.*
    A. It makes the heart the issue, not just the behavior.
    B. It focuses correction on deeper things than changed behavior.
    C. It provides a opportunity to confront what is going on in the heart.
    D. It turns your concern to unmasking your child's sin, helping him to understand how it reflects a heart that has strayed.
    E. It leads to the cross of Christ.
    F. It underscores the need for a Savior.
    G. It provides opportunities to show the glories of God, Who sent His Son to change hearts and free people enslaved to sin. (p. 6)

8. *What is the fundamental tenet of this book?*
    The heart is the wellspring of life. (p. 6)

9. *What is the fundamental task of parenting?*
    The fundamental task of parenting is shepherding the hearts of your children. (p. 6)

Chapter Two

Your Child's Development: Shaping Influences

1. *Give a simple description of shaping influences.*
   Shaping influences are those events and circumstances in a child's developmental years that prove to be catalysts for making him the person he is. (p. 10)

2. *What do the major passages dealing with the family (Deut. 6; Eph. 6; and Col. 3) presuppose?*
   These passages presuppose the lifelong implications of early childhood experience. (p. 10)

3. *The person your child becomes is a product of what two things?*
   A. His life experience.
   B. How he interacts with that experience. (p. 10)

4. *List the six shaping influences suggested by the author.*
   A. Structure of family life
   B. Family values
   C. Family roles
   D. Family conflict resolution
   E. Family response to failure
   F. Family history (pp. 11–14)

5. *Cite a statement and/or question that best helps you understand each of the six shaping influences.*
   A. Structure of family life
      1. How are the parenting roles structured?
      2. Are there other children or is family life organized around only one child?
   B. Family values
      1. Do parents get more stressed over a hole in the child's school pants or a fight between schoolmates?
      2. Where does God fit into the family life? Is life organized around knowing and loving God or is the family in a different orbit than that?
   C. Family roles
      1. Is the father involved in every aspect of the family life?
      2. Things like who pays the bills or who makes family appointments say much about family roles.
   D. Family conflict resolution
      1. Does the family know how to talk about their problems?
      2. Do they resolve things, or do they simply walk away?
   E. Family response to failure
      1. Are children made to feel foolish when they fail?
      2. Some parents show a marvelous ability to see failed attempts as praiseworthy efforts.
   F. Family history
      1. Some family members enjoy good health while others must structure their lives around sickness or disease.
      2. Some families have deep roots in the neighborhood while others are up-rooted continually. (pp. 11–14)

6. *List and discuss the two mistakes made in interacting with the shaping influences of life.*
   A. The first mistake is seeing shaping influences deterministically. It is the error of assuming that the child is a helpless victim of the circumstances in which he was raised.
   B. The second mistake is denial. It is the mistake of saying the child is unaffected by his early childhood experience. (p. 15)

7. *Describe in one sentence the idea of "Christian determinism."*
   Child rearing is nothing more than providing the best possible shaping influences for your children. (p. 15)

Chapter Three

Your Child's Development: Godward Orientation

1. *What determines whether a child responds to rebuke and instruction as a mocker or a wise man? Cite references.*
   Proverbs 9:7–10—"It is the fear of the Lord that makes one wise and it is that wisdom that determines how he responds to correction." (p. 19)

2. *Because children are worshippers and they are never neutral, they either worship _____ or _____?*
   They worship either Jehovah or idols. (p. 19)

3. *In what sense does the author use the term "Godward orientation"?*
   In the language of Romans one, your children either respond to God by faith or they suppress the truth in unrighteousness. If they respond to God by faith they find fulfillment in knowing and serving God. If they suppress the truth in unrighteousness they will ultimately worship and serve the creation rather than the creator. (pp. 19–20)

4. *Cite and quote the two verses that teach the fact that children are never morally neutral, not even from birth.*
   A. Psalm 58:3—"Even from birth the wicked go astray; from the womb they are wayward and speak lies."

B. Psalm 51:5—"Surely I was sinful at birth, sinful from the time my mother conceived me." (p. 20)

5. *What does the author have in view when he discusses the subtle idols of the heart?*
Any manner of motives, desire, wants, goals, hopes, and expectations that rule the heart of a child are in view. (p. 21)

6. *Your children are not neutral. They respond to life in one of two ways. What are they?*
A. Either they respond to life as children of faith who know love and serve Jehovah; or,
B. They respond as children of foolishness, of unbelief, who neither know him nor serve Him. (p. 21)

7. *Your child is not just a product of those shaping influences. He interacts with all these things. Therefore, the story is not just the nature of the shaping influences of his life, but what?*
How he has responded to God in the context of those shaping influences (p. 23)

8. *Since it is the Godward orientation of your child's heart that determines his response to life, you may never conclude that his problems are simply what? Explain.*
You may never conclude his problems are a lack of maturity. Selfishness is not outgrown. Rebellion against authority is not outgrown. These things are not outgrown because they are not reflective of immaturity but of the idolatry of your child's heart. (p. 23)

9. *If man is only the sum total of the influences that shape him, what would have been the result of Joseph's experiences?*
He would have been a man that was bitter, cynical, resentful, and angry. (pp. 23–24)

10. *How do we explain Joseph?*
In the midst of difficult, shaping influences he entrusted himself to God. God made him a man who responded out of a living relationship with God. He loved God and found his orientation, not in the shaping influences of his life, but in the unfailing love and covenant mercies of God. (p. 24)

11. *In summary, what two issues must your parenting address?*
A. The shaping influences of your child's life.
B. Your child's Godward orientation. (pp. 24–25)

Chapter Four

You're In Charge

1. *If a parent is unsure about the nature and extent of his authority, his children will suffer in what ways?*
   A. They will never know what to expect from the parent because the ground rules will constantly be changing.
   B. They will never learn the absolutes and principles of God's Word that alone teach wisdom. (p. 27)

2. *When parents require obedience because they feel under pressure, obedience of children is reduced to what?*
   Obedience is reduced to parental convenience. (p. 27)

3. *For what reason do you as a parent have authority?*
   God calls you to be an authority in your child's life. You have the authority to act on behalf of God. (p. 28)

4. *Cite and quote three passages of Scripture that teach that parents are to act in God's behalf.*
   A. Genesis 18:19—"For I have chosen him, so that he will direct his children and his household after him to keep the way of the LORD by doing what is right and just, so that the LORD will bring about for Abraham what he has promised him."

   B. Deuteronomy 6:2—"...so that you, your children and their children after
      them may fear the LORD your God as long as you live by keeping all his de-
      crees and commands that I give you, and so that you may enjoy long life."
   C. Ephesians 6:4—"Fathers, do not exasperate your children; instead, bring
      them up in the training and instruction of the Lord." (p. 28)

5. *What is the implication to the fact that a parent is God's agent, acting in God's behalf?*
   The parent also is a person under authority. The child and the parent are in the
   same boat. The child and the parent are both under God's authority. They have
   differing roles but the same master. (p. 29)

6. *Understanding that you are God's agent as a parent, deals not only with the right
   to direct, but it also provides what?*
   It provides the mandate to act. A parent has no choice. A parent must engage his
   children. A parent is acting in obedience to God. It is the parent's duty. (p. 30)

7. *By way of observation, most parents to not understand the appropriateness and ne-
   cessity of being in charge in their child's life. They rather take the role of what?*
   They take the role of advisor. (p. 31)

8. *What happens when the parent takes the role of advisor?*
   The child is learning that he is the valid decision-maker. (p. 31)

9. *Some parents argue, "Children only learn to be decision-makers as parents allow
   them to make decisions. We want children to learn to make sound decisions." What
   important issue is missed in this argument?*
   This argument misses the most important issue. Children will learn to be good
   decision-makers as they observe faithful parents modeling and instructing wise
   direction and decision-making on their behalf. (p. 31)

10. *Our culture has reduced parenting to what? Give examples.*
    A. Providing care.
    B. Parents often see the task in these narrow terms: The child must have food,
       clothes, a bed, and some quality time. (p. 32)

11. *The task God has given you is a pervasive one. Please explain.*
    Training and shepherding is going on whenever you are with your children.
    Whether waking, walking, talking or resting you must be involved in helping your
    child to understand life himself and his needs from a biblical perspective (Deut.
    6:6–7). (p. 32)

12. *What will anger, when displayed during correction and discipline, not bring about?*
    Anger will not bring about biblical righteousness. (p. 34)

13. *Explain the difference in discipline being corrective and not punitive.*
    A. If correction orbits around the parent who has been offended, the focus will be venting anger or perhaps taking vengeance. The function is punitive.
    B. If, however, correction orbits around God as the one offended, the focus is restoration. The function is remedial—it is designed to move a child who has disobeyed God back to the path of obedience. It is corrective. (p. 36)

14. *Many parents who lack a biblical view of discipline tend to think of it as what?*
    Revenge—getting even with the children for what they did (p. 36)

15. *Explain what Hebrews 12 says about discipline not being punitive, but corrective.*
    Hebrews 12 calls discipline a word of encouragement that addresses sons. It says discipline is a sign of God's identification with us as our father. God disciplines us for our good that we might share in His holiness. It says that while discipline is not pleasant, but painful, it yields a harvest of righteousness and peace. (p. 36)

16. *Explain why the biblical idea of discipline is so hard to get ahold of.*
    We don't see ourselves as God's agents. We therefore correct our children when they irritate us. When their behavior doesn't irritate us, we don't correct them. Thus, our correction is not us rescuing our children from the path of danger, it is rather us airing our frustration. (p. 37)

17. *For what matters may we not discipline our children?*
    You may not discipline for mere matters of self-interest or personal convenience. (p. 37)

18. *To what must a parent's correction be tied? Please explain.*
    Your correction must be tied to the principles and absolutes of the Word of God. The issues of discipline are issues of character development and honoring God. It is God's nonnegotiable standard that fuels correction and discipline. (p. 37)

Chapter Five

Examining Your Goals

1. *List the seven unbiblical perspectives in establishing goals for children.*
   A. Developing special skills
   B. Psychological adjustment
   C. Saved children
   D. Family worship
   E. Well behaved children
   F. Good education
   G. Control (pp. 40–44)

2. *Under each of the seven unbiblical perspectives list one or two statements and/or questions cited by the author that help you understand each one better.*
   A. Developing special skills
      1. Will the child receive biblical instruction in an accurate self-image, sportsmanship, loyalty, poise, endurance, perseverance, friendship, integrity, rights, competition and respect for authority?
      2. Will true success depend on the skills which these activities teach?
   B. Psychological adjustment
      1. The psychological gurus promise to teach you how to build self-esteem in your children.

2. How can you teach your children to function in God's kingdom, where it is the servant who leads, if you teach them how to make the people in their world serve them?

C. Saved children

    1. Parents think if their child would get saved all the problems of living would be solved.

    2. The child's profession of faith in Christ does not change the basic issues of child rearing. The parents' goals are the same. The things the child is called to are the same. He requires the same training he required before.

D. Family worship

    1. Some parents are persuaded that the family which prays together, stays together so they determine to have daily Bible reading times.

    2. As valuable as family worship is, it is no substitute for true spirituality.

E. Well behaved children

    1. Every parent has faced the pressure to correct a son or daughter because others deemed it appropriate. If the parent acquiesces, his parenting focus becomes behavior. The burning issue becomes what others think rather than what God thinks.

    2. What happens to the child who is trained to do all the appropriate things? When being well-mannered is severed from biblical roots in servanthood, manners becomes a classy tool of manipulation.

F. Good education

    1. The parents' goal is seeing their child achieve academic awards and scholarly recognition.

    2. Unfortunately scores of disillusioned and broken people are thoroughly educated. It is possible to be well educated and still not understand life.

G. Control

    1. Some parents have no noble goal at all. They simply want to control their children. These parents want their children to mind, to behave, to be good, to be nice.

    2. The control is not directed toward specific character development objectives. The concern is personal convenience and public appearance. (pp. 40–44)

3. *What is it that helps us answer the three questions posed by the author in the middle of page 47?*
The familiar question of the shorter catechism answers these questions.
Q: What is the chief end of man?
A: Man's chief end is to glorify God and to enjoy Him forever. (p. 45)

4. *If you teach your children to use their abilities, aptitudes, talents, and intelligence to make their lives better without reference to God, what will result?*
   You turn your children away from God. (p. 45)

5. *If your objectives for your children are anything other than, "Man's chief end is to glorify God and enjoy Him forever," you teach them to function in what way?*
   You teach them to function in the culture on its own terms. (p. 45)

6. *List at least two practical ways a parent can teach their child to function in the culture on its own terms.*
   A. We pander to their desires and wishes.
   B. We teach them to find their soul's delight in going places and doing things.
   C. We attempt to satisfy their lust for excitement.
   D. We fill their young lives with distractions from God.
   E. We give them material things and take delight in their delight in possessions.
   (p. 45)

7. *Because the chief end of man is to glorify God and enjoy Him forever, what is the parents' objective in every context?*
   The parents' objective in every context must be to set a biblical worldview before their children. (p. 46)

8. *Give one example of a parent presenting an unbiblical objective.*
   Teaching the child to obey and to perform for approval from the parent and from others. (p. 46)

9. *Biblical counsel directs the child to whom and not to what?*
   Biblical counsel directs the child to God and not to his own resources. (p. 47)

Chapter Six

Reworking Your Goals

1. *Give three ways that the category of developing special skills can be focused toward a biblical worldview.*
   A. In a biblical worldview you should teach your children to exercise and care for their bodies as an expression of stewardship for God's gifts. Abilities should be developed because God has given the stewardship of talents and special capacities.
   B. Skills which would make your children more able to serve and open channels of ministry to others should be encouraged.
   C. Athletic activities can be a valuable way of providing family unity and oneness.
   D. Strenuous activity is valid to keep the body in excellent health. You must be concerned with strength and stamina for a life of service to God. (p. 50)

2. *Give at least three things that a child who has suffered an injustice could learn by being counseled from a biblical perspective.*
   A. He can learn to entrust himself to God in the face of unfair treatment.
   B. He should be exhorted to leave vengeance to God.
   C. He should learn to face injustice without retaliation. (p. 51)

3. *What two things must you always hold out to your children?*
   A. The need of Christ's invasive redemptive work.
   B. The child's obligation to repent of his sin and place his faith in Jesus Christ. (p. 52)

4. *Family worship is a means to what end?*
   Family worship is a means to knowing God. (p. 53)

5. *You need family worship that does what?*
   You need family worship that connects with your children and their lives. (p. 53)

6. *When you lose sight of the fact that the goal of family worship is knowing God, what happens?*
   When you lose sight of knowing God family worship becomes a family ritual. (p. 54)

7. *Teaching children "good behavior" without reference to God is essentially reduced to what?*
   It is simply an elaborate means of pleasant social manipulation. (p. 54)

8. *Describe manners or good behavior from a biblical perspective.*
   A. Manners are an expression and application of the duty of loving my neighbor as myself. It is a matter of teaching children to imitate the Lord Jesus' self-giving as set forth in Philippians 2.
   B. When saying "please" and "thank you" are rooted in understanding what it means to look out for the interests of others, they become expressions of biblical love.
   C. Waiting to eat until all are served is not just an empty social convention, it is a way of showing consideration for those around you. (p. 54)

9. *Since good grades are ultimately not your child's goal, describe where his focus needs to be.*
   What is important is that your child learn to do his work diligently for God. God has promised that He will reward the faithful. Knowing that gifts and abilities are a stewardship from the Lord, your child's objective should be faithfulness. (p. 55)

10. *Explain how holding out God's standard to your children and keeping before them His law can be a schoolmaster to take them to Christ.*
    Faced with being kind to one who abuses you, there is nowhere to go but to God, who alone can enable a person to respond in love. When your child's heart desires revenge, when she must love an enemy, when her faith demands she leave room for God's justice; there is no place to go but to the cross. She will not be able to embrace these things without embracing Christ. Thus you are always pointing to Christ and His work, power and grace. (pp. 55–56)

Chapter Seven

Discarding Unbiblical Methods

1. *What do the various unbiblical approaches to child rearing have in common?*
   The human mind is the standard. It may be our own mind—"There is nothing wrong with what my father did"—or it may be the mind of others—"Dr. 'So and So' on talk radio advocated this and it sounds good to me. . ." (p. 59)

2. *What is the point of the "I didn't turn out so bad" approach?*
   The point is that many parents unquestioningly employ whatever method their parents employed. When they correct their kids, they are simply echoing their parent's words and tone. (p. 60)

3. *Cite one method born out of pop psychology.*
   One method born out of pop psychology is bribery. (p. 60)

4. *What is the point of appeal in bribery?*
   The point of appeal in bribery is crass self-interest. (p. 61)

5. *With what are methods such as bribery concerned?*
   They are only concerned with instances of behavior. (p. 61)

6. *For what should children not be rewarded?*
   They should not be rewarded for fulfilling normal responsibilities. (p. 61)

7. *In behavior modification, to what is the heart trained? Explain.*
   The heart is trained to greed and selfish interests and to working for rewards. The point of appeal is to Junior's greed. Because Junior lives a lust driven life in which he will perform for ice cream and other goodies, the program seems to work. (p. 61)

8. *Cite two examples given by the author of the emotional method.*
   A. "It really makes me feel bad when you talk like that. You are hurting my feelings . . ."
   B. Another variety of emotional appeal is to shame a child. (p. 63)

9. *Give two examples of the punitive correction method.*
   A. The punishment may be being hit or yelled at.
   B. The punishment may be simple privation of something that the child desires. The attempt is to keep the child in control through the negative experience of punishment. (p. 64)

10. *Based on the illustration given by the author regarding grounding, what problem is caused by grounding? Explain.*
    Generally speaking, grounding does not deal with the issues that caused the poor behavior for which a child is being grounded. Grounding is not designed to do something for the child. It is designed to do something against him. Grounding is not corrective, it is simply punitive. It does not biblically deal with the issues of the heart that were reflected in the child's wrong behavior. (p. 64)

11. *According to the author, why is grounding so universally popular? Explain.*
    It is because it is easy. It doesn't require ongoing interaction. It does not require ongoing discussion. It does not assess what is going on inside the child. It does not require patient instruction and entreaty. Grounding is quick, incisive, simple. "You're grounded for a month. Go to your room." (pp. 64–65)

12. *Describe "Erratic Eclecticism."*
    A. It is erratic in that it moves about. There is no consistency.
    B. It is eclectic as it freely draws from many sources. The parent gets bits and pieces from a variety of methods. (p. 65)

13. *To what do these unbiblical methods lead? Explain.*
    A. They all lead to the same problems.
    B. They lead to superficial parenting, rather than shepherding the hearts of our children. They only address behavior. Hence they miss the point of biblical discipline. (p. 66)

14. *What does superficial parenting that never addresses the heart biblically produce?*
    It produces superficial children who do not understand what makes them tick. They must be trained how to understand and interpret their behavior in terms of heart motivation. If they never have that training they will drift through life never understanding the internal struggles that lie beneath their most consistent behavior. (p. 66)

15. *What are the experts actually telling you to do when they instruct you to find what works for each child?*
    They are saying that you must find the idols of the heart that will move this child. (p. 67)

16. *How does addressing only behavior in your children keep you from the cross of Christ? Explain.*
    It is impossible to get from preoccupation with behavior to the gospel. The gospel is not a message about doing new things. It is a message about being a new creature. It speaks to people as broken, fallen sinners who are in need of a new heart. (p. 67)

17. *Give two effects of using these unbiblical methods of discipline cited by the author in the middle of p. 68.* please confirm page #
    A. Character development is ignored. Children are not being trained to make ethical choices as responsible people living in reverence to God. They are learning how to jump through the parent's hoops and avoid the parent's displeasure. They learn to make choices based on expediency rather than principle.
    B. It produces distance between parent and child. Children soon see through the implicit and explicit manipulation. They eventually come to resent the crass attempts to control their behavior. They learn to play the cat-mouse game with you, but depth of relationship and communication is lost. (p. 68)

Chapter Eight

Embracing Biblical Methods—Communication

1. *What two elements must be woven together in a biblical approach to children?*
   A. One element is rich, full communication.
   B. The other element is the rod. (p. 71)

2. *Cite and quote the references where these two elements stand side by side. Also indicate in the quotation the words or phrases that suggest one or both of these methods.*
   Prov. 23:13–19—"Do not withhold discipline from a child; if you punish him with the rod, he will not die. ¹⁴Punish him with the rod and save his soul from death. ¹⁵My son, if your heart is wise, then my heart will be glad; ¹⁶my inmost being will rejoice when your lips speak what is right. ¹⁷Do not let your heart envy sinners, but always be zealous for the fear of the LORD. ¹⁸There is surely a future hope for you, and your hope will not be cut off. ¹⁹Listen, my son, and be wise, and keep your heart on the right path."
   Prov. 23:22—"Listen to your father, who gave you life, and do not despise your mother when she is old."
   Prov. 23:26—"My son, give me your heart, and let your eyes keep to my way." (p. 71)

3. *What does the use of the rod preserve?*
   The use of the rod preserves biblically rooted parental authority. God has given parents authority by calling them to act as his agents in child rearing. (p. 72)

4. *What does the emphasis on rich communication prohibit and/or provide?*
The emphasis on rich communication prohibits cold, tyrannical discipline. It provides a context for honest communication in which the child can be known and learn to know himself. It is sensitive but avoids a "touchy-feely" sentimentality. (p. 72)

5. *Discuss in three or four sentences the importance of communication being a dialogue and not a monologue.*
We often think of communication as the ability to express ourselves. Accordingly we think of ourselves as talking "to" our children. Instead you should seek to talk "with" your children. It is not only the ability to talk but the ability to listen. (p. 72)

6. *Cite and quote two passages that highlight the importance of listening.*
   A. Prov. 18:2—"A fool finds no pleasure in understanding but delights in airing his own opinions."
   B. Prov. 18:13—"He who answers before listening—that is his folly and his shame." (pp. 72–73)

7. *Your first objective in correction must not be to tell your children how you feel about what they have done or said. You must try to understand what is going on inside them. Give three questions suggested by the author that will help you do just that.*
   A. What is the specific content of the abundance of his heart in this circumstance?
   B. What was the temptation?
   C. What was his response to that temptation? (pp. 73–74)

8. *State in three simple propositions the objective of your communication, and then summarize them.*
   A. The behavior you see is a reflection of the abundance of your child's heart.
   B. You want to understand the specific content of the abundance of his heart.
   C. The internal issues of the heart are of greater import than the specifics of the behavior, since they drive behavior.
   In summary: You want to understand your child's inner struggles. You need to look at the world through his or her eyes. This will enable you to know what aspects of the life giving message of the gospel are appropriate for this conversation. (pp. 75–76)

9. *Explain why it would be difficult for a child to answer the question, "Why did you hit your sister?"*
He is simply being asked questions he cannot answer. He lacks the depth of understanding and self-reflection to be able to respond intelligently to his mother's

or father's questions. He needs to have the issues focused in a different way. (p. 78)

10. *List three or four questions that can get to the "why" issue in productive ways.*
    A. What were you feeling when you hit your sister?
    B. What had your sister done to make you mad?
    C. Help me understand how hitting her seemed to make things better.
    D. Help me understand how hitting her may seem to make things worse?
    E. What was the problem with what she was doing to you?
    F. In what other ways could you have responded?
    G. How do you think your response reflected trust or lack of trust in God's ability to provide for you? (p. 78)

11. *In what way can you stand both above and beside your child as you help him understand the internal struggles with his sin?*
    A. You are above him because God has called you to a role of discipline and correction.
    B. You are beside him because you, too, are a sinner who struggles with anger, etc. toward others. (p. 79)

Chapter Nine

Embracing Biblical Methods—Types of Communication

1. *In the author's opinion what is Paul's point in I Thessalonians 5:14?*
   1 Th 5:14—"And we urge you, brothers, warn those who are idle, encourage the timid, help the weak, be patient with everyone."
   Paul's point is that differing conditions in the hearer require differing forms of speaking. (p. 81)

2. *List three things that communication for the purpose of correction does.*
   A. Correction remedies something wrong.
   B. Correction gives your children insight into what is wrong and what may be done to correct the problem.
   C. Correction helps your children to understand God's standard and teaches them to assess their behavior against that standard. (p. 82)

3. *What does a rebuke do?*
   A rebuke censures behavior. (p. 83)

4. *Discuss "entreaty" in three to four sentences.*
   Entreaty is earnest and intense communication. It involves pleading, soliciting, urging and even begging. It is the earnest pleading of a father or mother who, understanding his child, the ways of God, and the extremity of the moment, is

willing to bare his soul in earnest pleading for his child to act in wisdom and faith. (p. 83)

5. *Define instruction.*
   Instruction is the process of providing a lesson, a precept, or information that will help your children to understand their world. (p. 84)

6. *Describe what warnings do.*
   Warnings put us on guard regarding a probable danger. It is merciful speech, for it is the equivalent of posting a sign informing motorists about a bridge that is out. A warning faithfully alerts us to danger while there is still time to escape un-harmed. (p. 85)

7. *A warning is simply a what? Cite an example.*
   A warning is simply a statement that A leads to B. For example, laziness leads to slavery. The person who is lazy will end up in some form of servitude. (p. 85)

8. *Discuss "teaching" in three to four sentences.*
   Teaching is the process of imparting knowledge. Teaching is causing someone to know something. Sometimes teaching takes place before it is needed. Often it is most powerfully done after a failure or problem. (p. 87)

9. *When will parents gain some of the most penetrating insights into their children?*
   Parents will gain insights into their children when they pray. Understanding what they pray and how they pray is often a window into their souls. (p. 87)

Chapter Ten

Embracing Biblical Methods—A Life of Communication

1. *For what does a regular habit of talking together prepare the way?*
   A regular habit of talking together prepares the way for talking in strained situations. You will never have the hearts of your children if you talk with them only when something has gone wrong. (p. 90)

2. *What is the best way to train your children to be active listeners?*
   The best way to train your children to be active listeners is by actively listening to them. (p. 90)

3. *Honest, thorough, truly biblical communication is expensive. List three of these expenses.*
   A. Time
   B. Physical and spiritual energy
   C. Mental stamina (pp. 90–91)

4. *List at least three ways that you must bring integrity to your interaction with your children.*
   A. Let them see sonship with the Father in you.
   B. Show them repentance.
   C. Acknowledge your joys and fears and how you find comfort in God.

    D. Live a shared life of repentance and thankfulness.

    E. Acknowledge your own sin and weakness.

    F. Admit when you are wrong.

    G. Be prepared to seek forgiveness for sinning against your children. (p. 91)

5. *The teen years are a time when the teen develops comradery with those who "understand them." The attraction the "wrong crowd" holds is not a license for being bad. What is the attraction of the "wrong crowd"? Explain.*
The attraction of the "wrong crowd" is comradery. Children long to be known, understood, discipled and loved. (p. 92)

6. *In the chart given by the author on page 93 what does influence represent?*
In this chart influence represents the willingness of a child to place himself under authority because of trust. (pp. 93–94)

7. *Give the author's description of communication.*
Communication is the art of expressing in godly ways what is in my heart and of hearing completely and understanding what another thinks and feels. (p. 95)

8. *There is a simple way to look at the cost of deep, full-orbed communication. Explain.*
You must regard parenting as one of your most important tasks while you have children at home. This is your calling. You must raise your children in the fear and admonition of the Lord. You cannot do so without investing yourselves in a life of sensitive communication in which you help them understand life and God's world. There is nothing more important. You have only a brief season of life to invest yourself in this task. (p. 97)

9. *Give some practical examples of the costs that you will incur in parenting.*
    A. Parenting will mean that you can't do all the things which you could otherwise do.

    B. It will affect your handicap at golf.

    C. It may mean your home does not look like a picture from *Better Homes and Gardens.*

    D. It will impact your career and ascent on the corporate ladder.

    E. It will alter the kind of friendships which you will be available to pursue. It will influence the kind of ministry you are able to pursue.

    F. It will modify the amount of time you have for bowling, hunting, television, or how many books you read.

    G. It will mean that you can't develop every interest that comes along. (p. 97)

Chapter Eleven

Embracing Biblical Methods—The Rod

1. *Why can a child's problem not be solved with only instruction and direction? Explain and give Scripture support.*
   If children are born ethically and morally neutral, then they do not need correction, they need direction. They do not need discipline, they need instruction. But children are not born morally and ethically neutral. The Bible teaches that the heart is "deceitful and desperately wicked" (Jeremiah 17:9, KJV). The child's problem is not an information deficit. His problem is that he is a sinner. (p. 101)

2. *The rod addresses what needs of the child? Explain and support with Scripture.*
   The rod is addressed to needs within the child. These needs cannot be met by mere talk. Proverbs 22:15 says, "Folly is bound up in the heart of a child, but the rod of discipline will drive it far from him." God says there is something wrong in the child's heart. Folly or foolishness is bound up in his heart. This folly must be removed, for it places the child at risk. (p. 102)

3. *Describe the rod used in its proper setting.*
   The rod is not a matter of an angry parent venting his wrath upon a small helpless child. The rod is a faithful parent, recognizing his child's dangerous state, employing a God-given remedy. The issue is not a parental insistence on being obeyed. The issue is the child's need to be rescued from death—the death that results from rebellion left unchallenged in the heart. (p. 103)

4. *Describe the results of properly administered discipline.*
   Properly administered discipline humbles the heart of a child, making him subject to parental instruction. An atmosphere is created in which instruction can be given. The spanking renders the child compliant and ready to receive life giving words. (p. 104)

5. *All children don't just learn to obey on their own. Cite and quote Scripture for this truth.*
   A. Proverbs 29:15—"The rod of correction imparts wisdom, but a child left to himself disgraces his mother."
   B. Proverbs 29:17—"Discipline your son, and he will give you peace; he will bring delight to your soul." (p. 104)

6. *You must use the rod if you are going to accomplish three things. What are they?*
   A. If you are going to rescue your children from death.
   B. If you are going to root out the folly that is bound up in their hearts.
   C. If you are going to impart wisdom, you must use the rod. (p. 104)

7. *What is the rod?*
   The rod is a parent, in faith toward God and faithfulness toward his or her children, undertaking the responsibility of careful, timely, measured and controlled use of physical punishment to underscore the importance of obeying God, thus rescuing the child from continuing in his foolishness until death. (p. 104)

8. *In what context is the use of the rod placed?*
   The use of the rod is placed in the protected context of the parent-child relationship. (p. 105)

9. *In what way is the use of the rod an act of faith?*
   God has mandated its use. The parent obeys, not because he perfectly understands how it works, but because God has commanded it. The use of the rod is a profound expression of confidence in God's wisdom and the excellency of His counsel. (p. 105)

10. *In what way is the rod an act of faithfulness toward the child?*
    It is an expression of love and commitment. (p. 105)

11. *In what way is the rod a responsibility?*
    It is the parent determining to obey. It is the parent as God's representative, undertaking, on God's behalf, what God has called him to do. (p. 106)

12. *Discuss the use of the rod as physical punishment.*

    The rod is never a venting of parental anger. It is not what the parent does when he is frustrated. It is not a response to feeling his child has made things hard for him. It is always measured and controlled. The parent knows the proper measure of severity for this particular child at this particular time. (p. 106)

13. *In what way is the use of the rod a rescue mission?*

    The child who needs a spanking has become distanced from his parents through disobedience. The spanking is designed to rescue the child from continuing in his foolishness. The rod underscores the importance of obeying God. (p. 106)

14. *What is the only reason for a child to obey mom and dad?*

    God commands it. Failure to obey mom and dad is, therefore, failure to obey God. This is the issue. (p. 106)

15. *Describe in one or two sentences each of the five distortions of the rod.*

    A. The biblical concept of the rod is not the right to unbridled temper. God nowhere gives parents the right to throw temper fits at their children.

    B. The biblical concept of the rod is not to hit our children whenever we wish. It is not the right to use physical force whenever and however one wishes.

    C. The biblical concept of the rod is not a way for parents to vent their frustration with their children. The rod is not a way for you to vent your pent-up rage and frustration.

    D. The biblical concept of the rod is not the parent exacting retribution for the child's wrong. It is not payment due.

    E. The biblical concept of the rod is not to be associated with anger. (pp. 107–108)

16. *What is it biblically that keeps a parent from spanking his child. Cite and quote Scripture.*

    A. Hatred is what will keep the parent from spanking his child. Love will force them to do it.

    B. Prov. 13:24—"He who spares the rod hates his son, but he who loves him is careful to discipline him." (p. 109)

17. *Cite and quote the scriptural response to the objection, "I am afraid it will make him rebellious and angry."*

    Proverbs 29:17—"Discipline your son, and he will give you peace; he will bring delight to your soul." (p. 109)

18. *Give four reasons why the rod "doesn't work."*
    A. Inconsistent use of the rod.
    B. Failure to persist.
    C. Failure to be effective.
    D. Doing it in anger. (pp. 110–111)

19. *List at least five benefits of the rod.*
    A. The rod teaches outcomes to behavior.
    B. The rod shows God's authority over mom and dad.
    C. The rod trains a child to be under authority.
    D. The rod demonstrates parental love and commitment.
    E. The rod yields a harvest of peace and righteousness.
    F. The rod returns the child to the place of blessing.
    G. The rod promotes an atmosphere of closeness and openness between parent
       and child. (pp. 111–113)

20. *Substantiate scripturally the fact that both communication and the rod are designed
    to work together.*
    Hebrews 12:5–6—"And you have forgotten that word of encouragement that ad-
    dresses you as sons: 'My son, do not make light of the Lord's discipline, and do
    not lose heart when he rebukes you, ⁶because the Lord disciplines those he loves,
    and he punishes everyone he accepts as a son.' " (p. 113)

21. *What does the use of the rod preserve?*
    Biblically rooted parental authority. (p. 113)

22. *What does the emphasis on rich communication prohibit?*
    Rich communication prohibits cold, tyrannical discipline. (p. 113)

23. *Give the non biblical distortions of the rod and communication.*
    A. The person who is comfortable with the rod can fall into the distortion of being
       authoritarian.
    B. A parent for whom communication is natural and easy may tend toward per-
       missiveness. (pp. 113–114)

Chapter Twelve

Embracing Biblical Methods—Appeal to the Conscience

1. *The God-given reasoning capacity that distinguishes issues of right and wrong is called what?*
   The reasoning capacity that distinguishes issues of right and wrong is the conscience. (p. 116)

2. *Because of a person's conscience his thoughts do one of two things. What are they?*
   They either or excuse or accuse. (p. 116)

3. *Discuss in three or four sentences the author's conclusions from the passage in Proverbs 23.*
   Proverbs 23 justifies the use of the rod in correction. The rod, however, is not the only instrument of training in the passage. There is another. It is an appeal to the conscience. Solomon is not soft on using the rod, but he realizes the limitations of using the rod. He knows that the rod gets the attention but the conscience must be plowed up and planted with the truth of God's ways. (p. 116)

4. *What is Christ's pattern as seen in the Matthew 21 passage?*
   Christ appeals to their conscience so they cannot escape the implications of their sin. Thus, He deals with the root problems, not just the surface issues. (p. 118)

5. *What should be the focal point of your discipline and correction? Explain.*
   The focal point of your discipline and correction must be your children seeing their utter inability to do the things which God requires unless they know the help and strength of God. Your correction must hold the standard of righteousness as high as God holds it. God's standard is correct behavior flowing from a heart that loves God and has God's glory as the sole purpose of life. This is not native to your children. (p. 120)

6. *What is the alternative to this focus on proper biblical discipline?*
   A. It is to reduce the standard to what may be fairly expected of your children without the grace of God.
   B. It is to give them a law they can keep.
   C. It is a lesser standard that does not require grace and does not cast them on Christ, but rather on their own resources. (p. 120)

7. *In what does dependence on their own resources result?*
   A. It moves them away from the cross.
   B. It moves them away from any self assessment that would force them to conclude that they desperately need Jesus' forgiveness and power. (pp. 120–121)

8. *What is the result of giving children a keepable law and telling them to be good?*
   The result is hypocrisy and self-righteousness. (p. 121)

9. *What is the genius of Phariseeism?*
   It reduced the law to a keepable standard of externals that any self-disciplined person could do. (p. 121)

10. *Why must correction and shepherding focus on Christ?*
    It is only in Christ that the child who has strayed and has experienced conviction of sin may find hope, forgiveness, salvation and power to live. (p. 121)

Chapter Thirteen

Shepherding the Heart Summarized

1. *Simply list the six key summary points given in chapter 13.*
   A. Your children are the product of two things.
   B. The heart determines behavior.
   C. You have authority because God has made you His agent.
   D. Since the chief end of man is to glorify God and enjoy Him forever, you must set such a world-view before your children.
   E. Biblical goals must be accomplished through biblical methods.
   F. God has given two methods for child-rearing. (pp. 122–123)

2. *Parenting involves what two things?*
   A. Providing the best shaping influences you can.
   B. The careful shepherding of your children's responses to those influences. (p. 122)

3. *You have authority because God has made you His agent. What does this mean?*
   This means you are on His errand, not yours. (p. 122)

4. *What two methods for child rearing has God given?*
   A. Communication
   B. The rod (p. 123)

Chapter Fourteen

Infancy to Childhood: Training Objectives

1. *What is the primary characteristic of this first stage of development?*
   The primary characteristic of this first stage of development is change. (p. 128)

2. *List the four areas of change cited by the author.*
   A. Physical
   B. Social
   C. Intellectual
   D. Spiritual (pp. 128–129)

3. *What is the most important lesson for the child to learn in this period?*
   He is an individual under authority. He has been made by God and has a responsibility to obey God in all things. (p. 129)

4. *Cite and quote the key passage of Scripture for this period.*
   Eph 6:1–3—"Children, obey your parents in the Lord, for this is right. ² 'Honor your father and mother'—which is the first commandment with a promise—³'that it may go well with you and that you may enjoy long life on the earth.' " (p. 129)

5. *To whom is obedience a response? Explain.*
   Obedience is a response to God. Children must learn that they have been made for God. They have a duty to Him. He has the right to rule them. They owe Him obedience. (p. 130)

6. *What will result if your children fail to see this truth?*
   Your children will never submit to you without this truth. They will never see living in terms of bringing glory to God. They will be self-absorbed—the prime objects of worship in their own world. (p. 130)

7. *What is a specific application of being a creature under God's authority?*
   A specific application is submission to earthly authority. (p. 130)

8. *What does submission to parents mean?*
   Submission to parents means honoring and obeying. (p. 131)

9. *What is the function of the rod and communication?*
   The function of the rod and communication is rescue. (p. 132)

10. *What does it mean to honor parents?*
    Honoring parents means to treat them with respect and esteem because of their position of authority. It is honoring them because of their role of authority. (p. 132)

11. *If a child is going to honor his parents it will be the result of what two things?*
    A. The parent must train him to do so.
    B. The parent must be honorable in his conduct and demeanor. (p. 132)

12. *What is one of the clearest ways to show honor to a parent?*
    One of the clearest ways to show honor is in the way children speak to their parents. (p. 132)

13. *What is obedience?*
    Obedience is the willing submission of one person to the authority of another. It means more than a child doing what he is told. It means doing what he is told; Without Challenge, Without Excuse, and Without Delay. (p. 134)

14. *Cite two or three examples of a way a parent trains his children unbiblically about obedience.*
    A. A parent may train them to obey only after they have yelled.
    B. A parent may train them to obey only if they wish to.

C. A parent may train them to obey after the parent has pleaded or threatened.
D. The parent may not train them to obey at all. (p. 134)

15. *How often should a parent allow his children to disobey without dealing with them?*
You should never allow your children to disobey without dealing with them. (p. 135)

16. *Obedience is not simply an issue between the parent and the child, but between the child and whom?*
Obedience is also between the child and God. (p. 136)

17. *Give three unacceptable responses when teaching your children to appeal to authority.*
A. You cannot accept refusal to obey.
B. You cannot accept obedience only when your children are convinced you are right or fair.
C. You cannot be required to sell them on the propriety of your directives. (p. 136)

18. *In what way is the appeal process a safety check for the parent?*
Perhaps the parent has spoken quickly without careful thought. Appeal provides a context for you to rescind a directive that was spoken in haste or was inappropriate. (p. 136)

19. *In what way is the appeal process a safety check for the child?*
The child knows that they have permission to appeal a parental directive. They know that mom and dad will honestly reconsider and will rescind their directive if that is good for the individual or family. (pp. 136–137)

20. *Give at least five benefits of the appeal procedure.*
A. The child has some recourse.
B. He learns to submit to authority in a context that is not arbitrary.
C. He learns to approach his superiors in a respectful manner.
D. The parent has the opportunity to rethink a decision.
E. The parent can change his mind in the context of respectful appeal, but not in the presence of blatant rebellion. (p. 138)

21. *Give at least two examples of submission a parent can provide for their children.*
A. Through biblical authority over your spouse (Dads).
B. Through submission to your spouse (Moms).
C. Through biblical submission to employers.

D. Through your relationship to the state and the church.

E. Through the ways you respond to your disappointments with your authorities in the society, at the job and in the church; this teaches your children how to be under authority.

F. Through the attitudes you display; this teaches either biblical submission or unbiblical independence and rebellion. (p. 138)

22. *Training a child to do what he ought, regardless of how he feels, prepares him to be what?*

Training a child to do what he ought, regardless of how he feels, prepares him to be a person who lives by principle rather than mood or impulse. (p. 140)

Chapter Fifteen

Infancy to Childhood: Training Procedures

1. *What sends mixed messages to the child? Explain.*
   Disobedience coupled with failure to discipline sends mixed messages to the child. On the one hand you say they must obey. You tell them that temporal and eternal well-being is attached to obedience. On the other hand, you accept disobedience and tolerate behavior that places them at risk. (p. 144)

2. *When does a child need a spanking?*
   When you have given a directive that he has heard and is within his capacity to understand and he has not obeyed without challenge, without excuse or without delay, he needs a spanking. (p. 145)

3. *In what way does the parent fail if the parent fails to spank?*
   The parent fails to take God's Word seriously. (p. 145)

4. *What does inconsistency in spanking mean?*
   It means that correction revolves around your convenience rather than around objective biblical principle. (p. 145)

5. *If you accept challenge, delay or excuses, you are not training in submission, but in what?*
   A. You are rather training your children how to manipulate authorities and live on the ragged edge of disobedience.
   B. You teach them to toss you an occasional bone of obedience to keep you at bay. (pp. 145–146)

6. *List the eight suggested steps by the author for the "how" of spanking.*
   A. Take your child to a private place where he can be spoken with in privacy.
   B. Tell him specifically what he has done or failed to do.
   C. Secure an acknowledgment from the child of what he has done.
   D. Remind him that the function of the spanking is not venting your frustration or because you are angry, but to restore him to the place in which God has promised blessing.
   E. Tell the child how many swats he will receive.
   F. Remove his drawers so that the spanking is not lost in the padding of his pants.
   G. After you have spanked, take the child up on your lap and hug him, telling him how much you love him, how much it grieves you to spank him and how you hope that it will not be necessary again.
   H. Pray with him. (pp. 146–150)

7. *What must the spanking reflect?*
   The spanking must reflect your obedience to God's directives and concern for his good. Anything else is simply beating up on your child. (p. 147)

8. *When is a good time to press the claims of the gospel with your children?*
   A good time to press the claims of the gospel is when your children are being confronted with their need of Christ's grace and power during discipline. When the wax is soft during discipline the time is right to impress the glories of Christ's redemption. (pp. 149–150)

9. *Why do you spank?*
   You spank because God commands it. (p. 153)   please confirm page #

10. *What is the goal of correction?*
    To bring the child to sweet, harmonious, and humble heart submission to God's will that he obey Mom and Dad. (p. 150)

11. *When is a child old enough to be disciplined?*
    When a child is old enough to resist the parent's directives he is old enough to be disciplined. (p. 151)

12. *What is the parent tempted to do?*
    The parent will be tempted to wait until his children are speaking and able to articulate their rebellion before he deals with it. (p. 152)

13. *What could be the problem if a parent thinks, "If I follow your counsel all I'll do is spank"?*
    It could be that the parent is confronted with disobedience all day and tolerates it. As long as the parent is unwilling to require precision in obedience he or she will have sloppy responses to his or her directives. Consistency is the key. (p. 154)

14. *If discipline seems to not be working, what must the parent be prepared to do?*
    The parent needs to be prepared to be obedient to God whether or not it seems to bear fruit immediately. (p. 157)

15. *What explanations does the author give if discipline seems to not work.*
    Either there is a failure to be consistent in discipline or there is some basic lack of integrity in the parent's relationship with God, his child, or both. (p. 157)

16. *Simply list the six suggestions given by the author to recover lost ground in the area of discipline.*
    A. Sit down with your children and explain your new insights. Tell them what you believe you have done wrong in raising them.
    B. Seek their forgiveness for your failures as a parent.
    C. Give them specific direction about what changes you think are needed in their behavior, attitudes and so forth.
    D. Determine how you will respond to disobedience in the future.
    E. No new approaches can be successfully undertaken for the sole purpose of changing your children.
    F. Whatever you do will require patience. (p. 158)

17. *Your focus in recovering lost ground cannot be how to get your kids in line, but what?*
    Your focus must be what it means for you to honor God in your family life. (p. 159)

Chapter Sixteen

Childhood: Training Objectives

1. *The author uses the word "childhood" to refer to what chronological age group?*
   It is ages five to twelve. It is the elementary school years. (pp. 161–162)

2. *By way of review, what should each child learn at stage one?*
   A. He has come to see himself as a creature made by God, for God.
   B. He has come to understand what it means to be under authority.
   C. He has learned to obey, without challenge, without excuse, without delay. (p. 162)

3. *What is the issue during these middle years?*
   Character is the big issue during these middle years. (p. 162)

4. *At stage one the focus was obedience. About what three things were you concerned at that stage?*
   A. You were concerned with rooting out the native rebellion of your child's heart.
   B. You were concerned that he confront the natural tendency to resist authority.
   C. Thus, you addressed defiance and called your child to submission to the authority of God. (p. 163)

5. *The "make more rules" approach is an honest attempt to govern family life without what?*
   It is an honest attempt to govern family life without addressing character issues. It seems more manageable to generate rules than address behavior. (p. 164)

6. *To structure things around rules is to produce what?*
   You then produce children who learn to keep the rules. They become smug and self-righteous. They become modern pharisees whose cup is washed and clean on the outside, but filthy on the inside. (p. 165) please confirm page #

7. *What are the three perspectives on your child?*
   A. The child in relationship to God.
   B. The child in relationship to himself.
   C. The child in relationship to others. (pp. 166–169)

8. *Under each of the three categories listed above cite at least three questions indicated by the author as a way to determine your child's relationship in each one of these areas.*
   A. The child in relationship to God
      1. Is he concerned to know and love God?
      2. Is there any evidence that he is carrying on an independent (from you as a parent) relationship with God?
      3. Does he ever talk about God?
      4. How does he talk about God?
   B. The child in relationship to himself
      1. How does your child think about himself?
      2. How well does he understand himself?
      3. How aware is he of his strengths and weaknesses?
      4. Is he able to stick to a task without external props?
      5. Is he dependent upon the approbation of others or is he more self-possessed?
   C. The child in his relationship to others
      1. How does he interact with others?
      2. What sort of relationships does he have?
      3. What does he bring out in others?
      4. Does he fawn for the attention of others?
      5. Is he pleasant with other children his age? (pp. 166–169)

Chapter Seventeen

Childhood: Training Procedures

1. *What are some of the typical responses to the "two children, one toy" scenario?*
   A. Most ask who had the toy first, reducing it to an issue of justice.
   B. Some will holler for the children to "share" or "be nice."
   C. Some parents get out the timer. "OK, you get it for ten minutes and then your brother gets it for ten minutes."
   D. Some disregard the screaming, persuaded that children will fight less if their fights are ignored.
   E. Still others console themselves with the time worn idea that all brothers and sisters fight, therefore it is something they will outgrow. (p. 171)

2. *In the "two children, one toy" scenario, what are three appeals you cannot make? Explain.*
   A. You can't simply appeal to the physical—"Do you want a spanking?"
   B. You can't simply appeal to the emotions—"I don't like you when you . . ." or, "you hurt my feelings when you . . ."
   C. You cannot simply address their love of things—"Do you want me to take your toys away from you?" None of these approaches produce lasting fruit because they do not address the heart. (p. 172)

3. *Behavior has a "when", a "what", and a "why". Explain each.*
   A. The "when" describes the circumstances in which the behavior occurred.
   B. The "what" describes the things that were said or done.
   C. The "why" describes the internal heart issues that pushed or pulled the specific behavior. (p. 172)

4. *If you make your appeal to the conscience you avoid what? Explain.*
   If you make your appeal to the conscience you avoid making correction a contest between you and your child. Your child's controversy is always with God. (p. 175)

5. *Dealing with children by appealing to the conscience avoids what?*
   Dealing with children by appealing to the conscience avoids giving them a keepable standard so that they feel smug and righteous. They are faced with God's ways and how much they need the radical, renovating work of Christ. (p. 175)

6. *Character could be defined as living consistently with who God is and who I am. As a parent, you want to hold out who God is to your child as a basis for what?*
   You want to hold out who God is as a basis for making choices about what he should do and be. (p. 176)

7. *If you do not call your child to be what God has called him to be, you will end up doing what? Explain.*
   You will end up giving him a standard of performance that is within the realm of his native abilities apart from grace. It is a standard that does not require knowing and trusting God. It, therefore, drives him away from God rather than to God. In other words, you either call your children to be what they cannot be apart from grace, or you reduce the standard, giving them one they can keep. If you do that, you reduce their need for God accordingly. (p. 177)

8. *Reading the Proverbs daily provides a very natural setting for discussing moral purity. Explain.*
   In Proverbs 5 there is an extended discussion of moral impurity and its fruit as well as the benefits and sexual delights of purity. The passage warns freely about the danger of becoming ensnared and bound by the cords of sin. (p. 178)

9. *What other passage in Proverbs provides a context for frank discussion of sexuality?*
   Proverbs 7. (p. 179)

10. *Parents tend to see their children's behavior in very naive terms. Explain by citing the illustration used by the author.*

    Parents see the fight over a toy as simply a fight over a toy, when actually it is a failure to prefer others. It is selfishness. It is saying to others, "I don't care about what your wishes are, I want to have what I want." It is determination to live in the world in a way that exploits every opportunity to serve oneself. (p. 180)

Chapter Eighteen

Teenagers:
Training Objectives

1. *What are the benchmarks for this period of life?*
   The benchmarks for this period of life are the onset of puberty and the time when the child leaves home to establish a home of his own. (p. 184)

2. *The author cites several issues encountered by the teen during this period of life. Give at least three.*
   A. The teen years are years of monumental insecurity. He is neither a child nor an adult.
   B. Teens feel vulnerable about everything.
      1. They worry about their appearance.
      2. Do they have the right clothes?
      3. Are they wearing them right?
      4. What will their friends think about this shirt, dress, or new haircut?
   C. They feel anxiety about their understanding of life.
   D. They are unstable in the world of ideas.
   E. Teens feel insecure about their bodies.
   F. Teenagers experience apprehension about their personality. (pp. 184–185)

3. *Give three issues to which parents often attribute rebellion.*
   A. The fact the family had moved.

B. Their kids took up with new friends.
C. They started listening to heavy-metal music. (p. 185)

4. *Why does a rebellious teen easily find fellow rebels?*
   The teen falls in with rebellious company because he is a rebel, he does not become a rebel because of the company he keeps. (p. 186)

5. *Cite and quote the passage of Scripture that furnishes the parent with parenting goals for this period of life.*
   Proverbs 1:7–19—"The fear of the LORD is the beginning of knowledge, but fools despise wisdom and discipline. ⁸Listen, my son, to your father's instruction and do not forsake your mother's teaching. ⁹They will be a garland to grace your head and a chain to adorn your neck. ¹⁰My son, if sinners entice you, do not give in to them. ¹¹If they say, "Come along with us; let's lie in wait for someone's blood, let's waylay some harmless soul; ¹²Let's swallow them alive, like the grave, and whole, like those who go down to the pit; ¹³we will get all sorts of valuable things and fill our houses with plunder; ¹⁴throw in your lot with us, and we will share a common purse"—¹⁵my son, do not go along with them, do not set foot on their paths; ¹⁶for their feet rush into sin, they are swift to shed blood. ¹⁷How useless to spread a net in full view of all the birds! ¹⁸These men lie in wait for their own blood; they waylay only themselves! ¹⁹Such is the end of all who go after ill-gotten gain; it takes away the lives of those who get it." (p. 187)

6. *Give the three foundations for life citing specific verses for each.*
   A. The fear of the Lord—Proverbs 1:7
   B. Adherence to parental instruction—Proverbs 1:8–9
   C. Disassociation from the wicked—Proverbs 1:10–19 (pp. 188–195)

7. *Because everyone has a godward orientation he either worships whom or what?*
   Everyone worships either God or idols. (p. 188)   please confirm page #

8. *Since the question is not IF but WHAT your child will worship, what must you do?*
   You must freely confront him with the irrationality of worshiping any lesser god. (p. 187)

9. *Living in the fear of God means what? Explain.*
   Living in the fear of God means living in the realization of accountability to Him. It is living in the light of the fact that He is God and your teen is a creature. He sees all; everything is open before Him. Living in godly fear means living in full light of God as a holy God who calls His people to holiness. (p. 187)

10. *In learning the fear of God, the key to growth is not the cognitive identification of truth but what? Explain.*

It is understanding the pertinence of that truth in daily life. You and your children must understand the fear of the Lord in a manner that reorganizes your lives. (p. 188)

11. *You must make the fear of God functional in regular living. Cite the example given by the author and also the solution parents must provide.*

A. The example—Teenagers struggle with the fear of man. They worry about what their friends will think of them. They make decisions based on fearing the disapprobation of their peers.

B. Parental solution—You have to talk with them, helping them to see the ways they are experiencing the fear of man. Then, you must help them understand the bondage that is produced by living for the approval of others. Help them see the futility and idolatry of organizing life around the desire to have approbation. (p. 188)

12. *What vision does Proverbs 1:8–9 hold out?*

Proverbs 1:8–9 holds out a vision of children seeing in their parents a source of wisdom and instruction. It asserts that children will be enriched and greatly benefitted by adherence to the values and instruction of their parents. (p. 190)

13. *Give at least five reasons the parent should be more relevant to his children than anyone else.*

A. You know them.
B. You know the subtle nuances of their personalities.
C. You know their strengths and weaknesses.
D. You know their life experiences.
E. You understand them.
F. You also know God.
G. You know the Word of God.
H. You know the ways of God.
I. You have struggled and battled to live the Christian life.
J. You understand the disciplines and dangers of Christian living.
K. You understand the world in which they live.
L. You understand the pressures they are now facing.
M. You are committed to them and to God.
N. There is no one who loves them more, who is more deeply committed to them, who accepts them unconditionally.
O. There is no one who will be more honest or more tender. (pp. 190–191)

14. *If certain things are in place, your child will not generally want to remove himself from parental instruction. What are they?*
    A. Your relationship with your children must be honest.
    B. You must never give advice that suits your convenience or which spares you trouble or embarrassment.
    C. You must be parents that have demonstrated that you are not using them in any way. (p. 191)

15. *What is the primary context for parental instruction?*
    A. It is set forth in Deuteronomy 6.
    B. It is the ordinary context of daily living. (p. 192)

16. *What is the pitch to the young person in Proverbs 1?*
    It is the belonging. The attraction of giving in to the wicked comradery. The appeal is to a very human need to share mutuality with others. Your kids need to belong. (p. 194)

17. *What is the most powerful way to keep your children from being attracted by the offers of comradery from the wicked?*
    It is to make home an attractive place to be. (p. 194)

Chapter Nineteen

Teenagers:
Training Procedures

1. *Give five key summary thoughts, which if practiced by parents, will help them realize their goal of seeing their children come to know God.*
   A. Shepherding their hearts
   B. Appealing to their conscience
   C. Getting under the skin in correction and discipline
   D. Addressing the heart as the spring of life
   E. Refusing to give them a keepable standard that would eliminate their need of Christ. (p. 198)

2. *Explain what authority and influence are based on from the chart on page 202.*
   A. Authority in this chart denotes what may be accomplished with your child because you are stronger, faster, larger, and so forth.
   B. Influence represents the willingness of your child to place himself under your authority because they trust you. Your role as an influence is one of helping him to know his needs and be honest with himself. (p. 201)

3. *What are parents sometimes tempted to do when their children have questions? Cite examples.*
   A. Panic
   B. They respond with things like,

1. "I can't believe you are doubting God."
2. "You just have to believe."
3. "It is best not to question those things." (p. 204)

4. *What are some things that parents may have to do in helping their teens through the period of doubt?*
   A. You will sometimes have to help teens find answers to problems that you have never found difficult.
   B. You may need to educate yourself.
   C. You may have to help them locate books or other apologetic materials.
   D. You can share your own experience of dealing with questions of faith.
   E. You can show them that non-Christian philosophy is devoid of satisfying and unified answers to the major philosophical questions about humankind and the cosmos. (p. 204)

5. *What objective should your interaction with your child have?*
   Your interaction should have the objective of ministry. Be a constructive force in the life of your child. You want to be a source of encouragement and inspiration. (pp. 204–205)

6. *Because teenagers experience frequent failure, what must Christian parents become adept at doing?*
   As Christian parents you must become adept at taking your child to the cross to find forgiveness and power to live. (p. 206)

7. *What is a good metaphor for the parent and teenage child relationship?*
   It is the relationship that adults would have with one another. (p. 206)

8. *In an adult relationship you do not nitpick your friends over every little thing that needs attention, but you rather do what?*
   You look for broad themes of response. You try to understand the patterns of response and that's what you talk about. (p. 207)

9. *What does the author mean by the statement, "Your children need to develop the ability to think 'Christianly' "?*
   They need to learn to dissect any area of thought and subject it to biblical critique. (p. 208)

10. *What does it mean to discover and develop their peculiar ministry niche?*
    This involves understanding how God has equipped them to contribute to His people. It will also entail a deepening sense of mutuality with others and becoming established corporately with the people of God. (p. 209)

11. *God intends for the parenting task to be a temporary one. In the final analysis you must do what?*
    You must entrust your children to God. (p. 210)